Charles Ekin

Potable Water

How to Form a Judgment

Charles Ekin

Potable Water
How to Form a Judgment

ISBN/EAN: 9783744666459

Printed in Europe, USA, Canada, Australia, Japan

Cover: Foto ©ninafisch / pixelio.de

More available books at **www.hansebooks.com**

POTABLE WATER.

HOW TO FORM A JUDGMENT

ON THE

SUITABLENESS OF WATER FOR DRINKING PURPOSES.

ADDRESSED TO MEDICAL OFFICERS OF HEALTH, AND SANITARY AUTHORITIES, ETC.

BY

CHARLES EKIN,

FELLOW OF THE CHEMICAL SOCIETY.

SECOND EDITION.

LONDON:

J. & A. CHURCHILL, NEW BURLINGTON STREET.

1880.

PREFACE

TO THE

SECOND EDITION.

SINCE the publication of the first edition, the views I have ventured to put forward, as to the fallacy of judging chiefly of the wholesomeness of drinking water by the amount of organic matter it may contain, have received unexpected confirmation from no less an authority than Prof. Huxley, who, at a discussion at a recent meeting of the Chemical Society, gave it as his opinion, speaking as a biologist, " that a water may be as pure as can be as regards chemical analysis, and yet as regards the human body be as deadly as prussic acid; and, on the other hand, may be chemically gross and yet do no harm to anyone." "I am aware," continued he, " that chemists may consider this as a terrible conclusion, but it is true, and if the public are guided by percentages alone they may often be led astray. The real value of a determination of the quantity of organic impurity in a water is, that by it a very shrewd notion can be obtained as to what has had access to that water."

This opinion, so tersely and forcibly expressed, accords

entirely with the results of my experience, and is in strict conformity with what may fairly be called the common sense view of the subject, as I have endeavoured to show in the following pages.

C. E.

September, 1880.

WHAT CONSTITUTES POTABLE WATER?

THE difference of opinion that unfortunately exists amongst analysts of undoubted eminence with reference to what may or may not be pronounced a fit water for drinking purposes forms the *raison d'etre* of this *brochure*. That this difference exists widely, and threatens to become still more marked, is assumed to be within the knowledge of those to whom these pages are addressed, as there are few people interested in the health of the community who have not experienced the inconveniences, resulting often in a dead-lock, that arise from it.

Now that the Public-Health Act has conferred powers on Sanitary Authorities to institute proceedings with a view to closing impure wells and other sources of supply, and has left the decision to the local magistrates, it becomes more than ever desirable that some standard should be set up as a guide in such matters. The bench of magistrates listening to the conflicting statements of experts is like a rudderless ship at sea, without any exact knowledge to guide their decisions, or data upon which to form an opinion. It is hoped and believed that a consideration of the question conceived in an unbiassed spirit may tend to reduce order out of chaos, and that here as in most other things common-sense will come largely to our aid.

A practical experience afforded by the analysis of nearly two thousand samples of water is not so much put forward by the writer as a reason and proof of his ability to deal with this question with a view to its elucidation, as the fact that in a large number of cases he has had the opportunity of personally investigating the conditions under which the waters were collected; and further, that owing to the kindness of medical friends, he has enjoyed ample opportunities of examining waters that have given rise to enteric fever and other hardly less serious disorders. He has had, too, the good fortune to practise as an analyst in a district where, within a radius of 30 miles, every geological formation from the Chalk down to the Silurian is represented, and has thus had considerable experience of the diversities in the composition of water taken from the various strata.

The arguments in favour of this or that view have hitherto been conducted too much on *a priori* lines and an attack on the position from the other side,—an appeal to experience as opposed to mere anticipation,—will show us that pet theories are not only not always supported by facts, but must sometimes be very much modified by them.

It is not proposed to enter into the consideration of any technical details relating to water analysis and happily it is unnecessary. The processes by which chemists arrive at their results, and which during the last few years have been much improved in the direction of extreme accuracy, are not the subject of variance, with one notable exception however, viz: —that of the estimation of organic matter. Of the several methods in use for the estimation of organic matter, each is vaunted by its originator, as being the best and only reliable one, and the only agreement that seems so far possible amongst analysts (though here it must be admitted the unanimity is complete), is in decrying every other person's process.

Notwithstanding this exception, as we shall see further on, the general conclusions that have been arrived at are in no way affected. The facts then, so to speak, in connection with water analysis are not the subject of dispute, but the deductions to be derived from the facts; and here we enter a region which is altogether outside the province of a chemist pure and simple, his usurpation to the contrary notwithstanding, and the question becomes one rather for the medical expert. The chemist has no special knowledge or experience, beyond that pertaining to all intelligent educated men who take an interest in sanitary matters, to guide him in forming an opinion as to what may or may not be the conditions under which diseases may arise that are the outcome of unwholesome surroundings, and the sooner this is recognised and the matter relegated, in disputed cases, to those who are alone competent to give an authoritative opinion, viz:—those, who, practising medicine have made hygiene a special study, so much the better will it be for the health of the community.

In order to properly understand the subject it will be well to take a brief review of the various sources from which we take our water supplies.

To begin with rain water. This as being distilled from the clouds one would naturally expect to be as free from impurities as it is possible to obtain water: as a matter of fact however it ranks amongst the more impure supplies. Rain falling in the neighbourhood of dwellings and cultivated land washes out from the air the impurities, the result of emanations from the earth, which exist there, and is collected too on surfaces, such as roofs, which are in themselves more or less dirty. The Rivers Pollution Commissioners calculate that " half a pint of rain water often condenses out of about 3373 cubic feet of air, and thus in drinking a tumbler of such water, impurities, which would only gain access to the lungs in about 8 days, are swallowed at once," and they are of opinion, " that it is in vain to look to the atmosphere for a supply of water pure enough for dietetic purposes."

§

In the absence, however, of any evidence that such water is positively unwholesome, one is inclined to regard this con-demnation as too absolute. It would be nearer the truth to say that although at the best but a vapid and uninviting fluid, its use, failing better sources of supply, may be tolerated; always supposing of course that it is so stored as to render contamination by sewage impossible.

In the case of a country district, known to the writer, which is entirely dependent on rain for its water supply, he has beer unable, in spite of diligent inquiry into the history of the place, to trace any sickness to its use, and has not hesitated to allow his own family to drink the water there for many weeks together.

Rain falling upon the vast tracts of more or less unculti-vated uplands, which form the gathering grounds of so many of our lakes and rivers, is naturally less contaminated in the first instance, and has much of what organic matter it might have contained taken up by the herbage over which it passes, and thus gives rise to many supplies of undoubted purity. Loch Katrine which supplies Glasgow, the lakes of West-moreland and elsewhere, and many a rapid running river, afford instances that will at once occur to everyone. To these sources of supply may be added that of rivers generally where they have not become so fouled by manufacturing refuse and sewage as to render them unfit for human consumption. Rivers, which are fed by springs and rain water in the form of surface drainage, seem to have a self-purifying faculty, due partly to the subsidence of suspended impurity and partly to the agency of vegetation and of the vast army of organisms, identical with or allied to bacteria, which being endowed with various functions of reorganisation convert the carbon and nitrogen of organic matter into simpler inorganic compounds, these in turn to become the food of the more highly organised aquatic vegetation. As the poison of scarlet fever is disinfected and destroyed by free exposure to light and air, so it would appear that the poisonous germs which sometimes accompany sewage are destroyed by somewhat similar processes. Of course there are many rivers so impure as to be entirely unfit for human consumption, but there is no evidence that the health of towns that take in turn their water supply from such rivers as the Trent and Thames, and again pour their sewage into them, is injuriously affected by the use of such water; however repugnant and nasty the idea must be of drinking water that has been mixed with sewage, and however desirable it may be to obtain water, if possible, from purer sources.

Probably the purest drinking water is that obtained from springs, the purity being directly proportionate to the amount of surface impurity, and the more or less thorough percolation through porous strata. Lastly we come to wells, where water is collected by sinking holes in the earth to varying depths and which too yield water of greater or less purity as the conditions of the collection of the water are more or less favourable.

The water from shallow wells is, as a rule, very impure and gives rise to the large majority of cases of typhoid fever which occur in this country, and when we consider that it is computed that in Great Britain alone 200,000 suffer annually from this disease, of which number 20,000 die, it is hardly possible to over-rate the importance to a community of a proper water supply.

From this brief view of the sources from which we take our supplies, we pass to consider what the impurities are that affect water, how they may be estimated and what degree of purity we may reasonably expect a drinking-water to attain to. A very little consideration will show that absolute purity is hardly anywhere attainable, and in using the word it must be understood that it is meant only in a relative sense, which is however sufficient for all practical purposes.

All waters, rain water alone excepted, contain more or less mineral matter in solution from the soil with which they come in contact. Water like that of Loch Katrine, which has passed over surfaces more or less impermeable, contains the lowest proportion, while such water as is procured from a permeable formation, like the Chalk, contains a much larger proportion. It is a custom of some analysts to speak of the mineral constituents as "impurities," but inasmuch as in most cases these so-called impurities actually add to the wholesomeness of a water, this method of speaking is manifestly misleading. The mineral constituents add to the palatableness of drinking water, and except when present in too large quantities probably conduce to health by supplying what the system of the drinker requires.

We shall confine the word impurity then, to matters which are derived from the animal or vegetable world, and which are consequently spoken of as "organic." This organic matter may either be derived from the decay of vegetable matter, when it is comparatively harmless, or from animal matter, the result either of the direct mixing of sewage with the water, which constitutes the most dangerous form of contamination, or the water is fouled from its having been collected over an area where the surface is cultivated, and more or less heavily manured. I assume that it is proved beyond denial that this animal organic matter is highly dangerous to health. It is in itself highly putrescible, and probably sets up putrefactive changes in the system of the person drinking it. Further than this any human fæcal matter is also dangerous, inasmuch as it may contain the poison, call it germ or what you will, each infinitesimal particle of which is capable of setting up some special form of disease, such as typhoid or scarlet fever. It will easily be understood then, that the first and most important thing to do in analysing a sample of water that is used for drinking is to ascertain whether it contains any of this poisonous organic matter. Organic matter may be estimated roughly in a variety of ways. A water containing any appreciable amount when evaporated gives a coloured residue which when ignited, blackens, and gives off a more or less disagreeable odour. Secondly, this organic matter is readily oxidisable and may be roughly measured, proper precautions being taken, by the extent to which a solution of Potassium Permanganate of known strength is decolourised; or, thirdly, by using the same reagent under proper conditions, the organic matter is partially broken up with formation of ammonia, which ammonia can be collected and accurately determined, as little as one ten-thousandth part of a grain per gallon being readily recognisable. This process which was originated by Professor Wanklyn, and which is consequently identified with his name, is called by him the "albuminoid ammonia" process. Fourthly and lastly, we are indebted to the distinguished chemist Dr. Frankland, who has done so much by his labours as one of the Rivers Pollution Commissioners and otherwise, to advance this branch of his science, for a process for which he claims extreme delicacy by which the carbon and nitrogen of organic matter are separately determined.

Water containing sewage, when exposed to the air, or as it percolates through the soil, has the organic matter and ammonia it contains converted into nitrites, an intermediate stage of oxidation, and finally into nitrates, both these salts being in themselves harmless. These nitrates are held by Dr. Frankland to be evidence of " previous sewage contamination," and as such to be an objectionable element in a water, whereas Professor Wanklyn and his school " do not look upon the presence of considerable quantities of nitrates in water as any bar to its employment for domestic use," although they think that any water containing them should be exceptionally free from organic matter in order to be safe.*

Sewage also contains an appreciable quantity of chlorine in combination with alkalies or alkaline earths, and after deducting and making allowance for the amount of chlorine in combination which is dissolved out of the different strata through which the water passes, any excess of chlorine above this gives valuable indirect evidence of the amount of sewage contamination. In the immediate neighbourhood of the sea where much salt water is blown inland in the form of fine spray, and wherever there are natural deposits of salt the determination of the amount of chlorine becomes valueless, but generally speaking the proportion of chlorine throws important light upon the history of the water, so to speak, and in limited areas where the amount of chlorine present in unpolluted waters is exactly known it may be relied upon with confidence.

The amount of sewage in a water may therefore be measured directly by the amount of organic matter it contains as well as free ammonia which has escaped oxidation, and indirectly by the amount of nitrates, nitrites and chlorine.

Unfortunately we have no means by which animal may be distinguished from vegetable organic matter. It has been thought that the varying proportions of organic carbon and nitrogen as estimated by Dr. Frankland's process might throw some light on the subject, but it has failed, as a little reflection will show it must fail. The organic matter of sewage is of an albuminoid nature, and like the typical albumen of egg is coagulable by boiling. So too is much of the soluble matter of vegetation albuminous, the composition of both albumens, animal and vegetable, being identical. Ordinary herbage

* 'Water Analysis,' by Wanklyn and Chapman, p. 39.

contains a considerable per centage of albuminoids, and furnishes preformed the albumen required for the nourishment of the animals browsing on it.

The subject of the amount of vegetable organic matter in water has been carefully considered by the writer for many years.

It has been found in certain selected deep springs of undoubted purity as regards freedom from animal contamination, that at certain seasons, such as late autumn, and then especially when grass is abundant, the organic matter accompanied by ammonia has largely increased, whilst the nitrates and chlorine have remained quite stationary. The waters which are coloured even slightly with peat, and which form some of our best and largest supplies, are liable too to a considerable increase of nitrogenous organic matter, and have often been classed in consequence as waters of second-rate or doubtful . quality; and yet there has never been the slightest evidence, direct or indirect, of such waters having given rise to injurious effects,* and it is an abuse of language to speak of them as being in any way unwholesome. On the other hand it is quite a common thing to find shallow well waters, containing large amounts of nitrates, exceptionally free from organic matter. Waters which have undoubtedly given rise to typhoid fever have been found by the writer over and over again not to contain more than 0·05 parts of albuminoid ammonia in 1,000,000, and which notwithstanding their containing a large excess of nitrates have been passed by analysts of undoubted ability as being fit for drinking purposes. The attention of the writer was particularly drawn to this in the case of a

---

* Peat would seem in some cases to have a laxative effect, for new comers to a district supplied with water coloured by peat are said to be affected to a slight extent by simple diarrhœa, but this, even if proved to be really due to the water, soon passes off, and can in no sense be said to be injurious.

district where typhoid fever was hardly ever absent, and where the conditions were such as pointed exclusively to water as being the aggravating cause. The village in question with a population of over 1000 is situated on the table land of the great oolite, the land sloping away from it on its north and south sides. The porous rock on which the village is built is from 40 to 70 feet thick, and in this are sunk side by side the wells and privies. The consequence of this arrangement is that considered by itself the drainage is perfect. There is no pent up sewer gas, no nuisance of any kind, but as might be expected all the water is fouled. Owing to the kindness of the medical men practising in this district, whenever a case of typhoid fever occurred, an opportunity was given to analyse the water, with the result in many cases, as before stated, of finding the quantity of organic matter exceedingly small. The history of this district affords another instance of how prejudicially the differences of opinion amongst analysts sometimes operate. Within the last few years, steps were taken to have the whole of the down properly drained to prevent the pollution of the water. The authorities of the place had agreed after long years of hesitation to have this done, but prior to taking any steps it was thought necessary to take test samples from six different points in order to prove the water bad. The samples were taken where the pollution was evident, and analysed. Two only were found to contain an excess of albuminoid ammonia, but all contained a large excess of nitrates and were accordingly condemned. Before entering upon what would have been, for so comparatively small a community, a large outlay, it was thought desirable to have a second opinion and accordingly samples from the same six sources were sent to another analyst of repute. His figures were identical with those of the first analyst but inasmuch as in four cases the organic matter was small, he reported upon them as being fit for drinking purposes, and as a consequence of this difference of opinion the district in question remains undrained to this day.

The process of nitrification has lately been shown [*] to be something else than mere oxidation, the oxidation only taking place apparently in the presence of a distinct ferment, and this process of nitrification appears to take place with greater or less rapidity as the organic matter is more or less dangerous. The highly putrescible organic matter of sewage is liable to the most rapid change. In the case of the wells just referred to, where the water was only separated from the sewage depository by a few feet of very porous rock, the nitrification was so complete that, except in times of very heavy rainfall, hardly any organic matter escaped oxidation.

On the other hand in watching the test springs already referred to through a series of years, it was found that though the organic matter which must have been entirely of vegetable origin varied considerably in quantity, the nitrates varied so little as to give practically a constant figure.

Dr. Frankland has noticed the same thing. He says "whilst the oxidation of animal matters in solution in water yields abundance of nitrates and nitrites, vegetable matters furnish under like circumstances none, or mere traces of these compounds," and he comes to this conclusion from the results of his analysis of upland waters, which come in contact only with the vegetable matter of uncultivated soil, and which contain, if any, mere traces of nitrogen in the form of nitrates and nitrites.[†]

As has been already stated, it is on the value to be attached to the presence of excess of nitrates, that so much difference of opinion exists among analysts. Of the two rival schools, each of which has its distinguished leaders of well-known and

[*] Warington on Nitrification, 'Chemical Society's Journal,' vol. xxxiii, p. 44.

[†] 'Rivers Pollution Commission.' Sixth Report, p. 13.

tried men, one contends that inasmuch as nitrates are in themselves perfectly harmless salts, that in some cases they may be of prehistoric origin, *i. e.* derived from animal matter indeed, but which has been fossilised for countless ages, their presence or absence in a water is a matter of no significance. On the other hand, though it is allowed that nitrates are in themselves harmless, they are held to be a proof, inasmuch as they are the result of the oxidation of animal organic matter, of the water having been fouled by sewage, and they point to at least two dangers. Granted that the organic matter has become to a large extent oxidised and rendered harmless by the percolation through the soil of the water containing it, there is always the danger of the organic matter finding its way to the well or spring in an unoxidised, and therefore dangerous state, during periods of heavy rainfall. Although with a proper system of drainage a heavy rainfall acts beneficially by flushing sewers and carrying off accumulations of filth, it is a well-known fact that in villages and communities where the wells and privies and middens are sunk side by side in the earth, typhoid fever is almost always more rife in a wet season, the reason being that the organic matter is then carried too quickly to the well for it to be oxidised by contact with aërated and porous soil. The second danger is that we have no evidence that percolation through the soil, even if it has the power of rendering harmless the organic matter which may give rise to sporadic outbreaks of fever, has any effect on specific poisons (or germs). Indeed, the famous case of the Lausen epidemic, points to a directly contrary conclusion.*

* For a full account of this case see ' Deutsche Vierteljahrsschrift für öffentliche Gesundheitspflege,' vol. vi, p. 154. Briefly it is this :—A severe outbreak of typhoid fever broke out in Lausen, in the Canton of Basel, in August, 1872. The public water supply was a spring rising at the foot of a mountain (the Stockhalden), which was received into a sealed reservoir, and so conveyed to Lausen, that any pollution by the way or at its source was out of the question. Suspicion attached itself to the public supply, as

With reference to the derivation of nitrates from fossils, the writer would be the last to deny its possibility, as, so far as he knows, he is the only one who has ever published results showing that fossils do yield nitrates.* Nitric acid is also formed in the air to an appreciable extent, especially during thunder storms, and allowances must always be made for nitrates from these two sources, but practically the amount is always so infinitesimal as in no way really to influence the question.

Dr. Frankland calculates,† that 0·032 parts per 100,000 should always be deducted as representing the amount of nitrogen as ammonia, nitrites and nitrates, found in rain water. Manifestly the quantity must be very variable, but practically there can be no objection to this amount being taken as representing a fair average.

A little consideration will show that the custom of laying the chief stress on the amount of organic matter irrespective

it was found that all houses supplied from other sources were exempt from the attack. Investigation led to the discovery that cases of typhoid had occurred at a farm house in a valley, the other side of the Stock-halden, and the drainage from which farm went into a brook called the Furler. Finally it was also discovered that part of the stream lost itself in the Stockhalden, and after travelling for about a mile through the mountain, reappeared as the spring which forms the Lausen supply. Several hundredweights of salt were thrown into the stream, and salt was detected after a time in the Lausen spring, thus establishing the connection between the two. Then several hundredweights of flour were thrown in, but not a vestige appeared the other side of the mountain, showing the thoroughness of the percolation. The case, which is given at great length, and which was most elaborately investigated, proved beyond doubt that the fever poison was conveyed by water, and is interesting chiefly as showing that no amount of percolation, no matter how efficient, will keep back the typhoid poison.

* "Origin of Nitrates in Potable Water," 'Chemical Society's Journal,' March, 1871.

† 'Rivers Pollution Commission.' Sixth Report, p. 14.

of its origin is misleading and fallacious. Prof. Wanklyn states that all drinking waters should be required to be of such a degree of purity as not to yield more than $\frac{8}{100}$ parts per million of* albuminoid ammonia and as a type of water that is "vile and stinking" he gives a sample of dirty water taken from the Thames at London Bridge, which yielded $\frac{.50}{100}$ parts per million of albuminoid ammonia. It will be noticed that the amount of albuminoid ammonia is, therefore, only six times as much in very foul water as in a water that is wholesome.

If it contained only half as much again it would no longer be ranked as a first-class water.

Dr. Frankland too says, " Spring and deep well water ought not to contain in 100,000 parts more than 0·1 part of organic carbon or ·03 parts of organic nitrogen. If the organic carbon reaches 0·15 part in 100,000 parts, the water ought to be used only when a better supply is unattainable."† Thus, here also an increase of organic carbon from 1 part to $1\frac{1}{2}$ parts is sufficient to make the difference between a desirable or undesirable sample.

Dr. Tidy, who has ably vindicated the Permanganate process, considers that waters pure enough for drinking purposes should not require more oxygen to oxidise the organic matter present than from 0·05 to 0·15 part per 100,000 parts :—that if the amount rises to 0·21 part the water is of doubtful purity, and if above this the water is impure.

We have here then an instance, surely the only one of the kind on record, where half as much again makes all the difference between a dose that is safe and one that is unsafe. To put it in another way, in the case of an infected water, six typhoid germs are harmless whilst nine would be hurtful!

* ' Water Analysis,' p. 62.
† ' Rivers Pollution Commission.' Sixth Report, p. 426.

Frequent allusion having been made to the Rivers Pollution Commissioners' Report, it may be well at this point to refer more particularly to their work, as being an authoritative exposition by able men, selected by Government, it is to be presumed, for their special knowledge of the subject they had to deal with.

The Commission was appointed in 1868 to inquire into the best means of preventing the pollution of rivers, and incidentally into the water supply generally of the United Kingdom. The sixth and final report which embraces all the reports that had gone before, so far as the water supply is concerned, was published in 1874. All the analytical work was done in the laboratory of Dr. Frankland, himself one of the Commissioners, and in all 1274 samples of potable water were examined. This is the first attempt that has been made to deal with the subject on anything like an adequate scale, and the mass of facts thus brought together affords material for generalisation and serves amongst other useful purposes, as a *point d'appui* for fresh departures. The thoroughness of the work is worthy of all praise, but as might be anticipated from the necessarily hurried visits of the Commissioners to the various localities the report contains several errors, which however do not perhaps seriously affect its general value.

Unfortunately Dr. Frankland is the originator of a process for the estimation of organic matter, which is of course " the only one yielding results which are trustworthy."* The consequence is that a standard has been set up of organic purity as measured by this special process which has no foundation in fact, and which, therefore, just to the extent to which it has been relied upon, vitiates the general results and conclusions of the Report. The fatal error has been made of judging chiefly of the suitableness of water from the amount of organic matter it contains, *quite irrespective of the nature and origin of the*

* 'Rivers Pollution Commission.' Sixth Report, p. 5.

organic matter, so that many water supplies of undoubted wholesomeness have been condemned, whereas others of more than doubtful purity have been classed as unpolluted. Water from wells of a depth of 100 feet or more, containing as much as 3·5 parts per 100,000 of nitrogen as nitrates, and collected as in one case at the foot of a churchyard, is considered wholesome, on the ground that " the exhaustive filtration to which it has been subjected, in passing downwards through so great a thickness of material, and the rapid oxidation of the dissolved organic matter in a porous and aerated medium, afford considerable guarantee that all noxious constituents have been removed;" and yet the Commissioners quote at length the case of the Lausen Epidemic already referred to, in which it was found that percolation through soil to the depth of more than a mile was insufficient to remove sewage from water. Not only so, but so inconsistent are they in their conclusions, that in their article on the improvement of potable water by filtration, they go the length of saying "we desire it to be distinctly understood that, although the purification of water polluted by human excrements, may reasonably be considered on theoretical grounds to be some safeguard against the propagation of epidemic diseases, *there is not in the form of actual experience a tittle of trustworthy evidence* to support such a view. On the contrary, the investigation of the epidemic of typhoid fever at Lausen proves that *even very efficient filtration does not prevent the propagation of that fever by water.*"* The italics are ours.

A useful table on the average composition of potable waters is given by the Commissioners,† but this too is marred by conclusions drawn from insufficient data. For example, on the faith of only one sample of spring water taken from the Magnesian Limestone, it is stated that potable water from this

* Sixth Report, p. 221.
† Rivers Pollution Commission. Sixth Report, p. 131.

formation contains on an average as much as 1·686 parts in 100,000 of nitrogen as nitrates and nitrites, but if we turn to the results of the analysis of this water * we find it stated that "this sample of water had been previously polluted to such an extent as to mask its true character. It contained but a minute proportion of organic matter, although it exhibited so much evidence of previous contamination with animal matter as to relegate it to the class of suspicious waters;" and notwithstanding this very questionable character, the results of the analysis are headed in large type, "Unpolluted Spring water from Magnesian Limestone!"

Passing from general considerations, we will briefly recapitulate the conclusions that we think may now fairly be arrived at, and then proceed to state the standard that experience dictates may be relied upon.

First then with regard to organic matter. It may be estimated in a variety of ways. The advocates of various processes concern themselves chiefly, not only in praising their own particular method, but in demonstrating very elaborately the fallacy of every one else's method. We will be more impartial. A fair trial of the different processes leads to the conclusion that all are absolutely worthless, so far as distinguishing between organic matter that is dangerous, and organic matter that is innoxious is concerned, but that probably all may be relied upon as giving a rough approximation as to whether organic matter is present in excess or not. Possibly the most convenient process is that of Professor Wanklyn, and the most accurate that of Dr. Frankland, but as the latter is confessedly "both troublesome and tedious and requires considerable manipulative skill,"† and as the less simple the process, the more the chances of error are increased, even in the most skilled and careful hands, to this extent it

* 'Rivers Pollution Commission.' Sixth Report, p. 115.
† Ibid., p. 5.

is objectionable. As indications of excess or otherwise, the figures decided upon by the authors of the several processes, and given at page 20, may be accepted without question. As giving any indication, however, of the wholesomeness of a water, they are useless, because both vegetable and animal organic matter (the latter only being dangerous) yield organic carbon and nitrogen and albuminoid ammonia, and in proportions so nearly alike as to be practically undistinguishable. An excess of organic matter is not necessarily an objectionable feature in a drinking water, for many, of what are confessedly our best and purest supplies, frequently contain an excess of organic matter; but neither on the other hand is a minimum of organic matter necessarily a satisfactory feature, for water from wells, especially from shallow wells, and which has undeniably given rise to typhoid fever will frequently be found to contain only a minimum quantity.

Therefore the quantity of organic matter a water contains affords no guide to its wholesomeness, and to lay the chief stress on this ingredient, irrespective of other considerations, is as unscientific as it is eminently misleading.

Sewage and all animal fæcal matter mixed with water contain large quantities of putrescible organic matter and ammonia, but no nitrates. When allowed to stand, a process of fermentation goes on, and as this subsides, oxidation commences with the formation of nitrites and nitrates at the expense of the organic matter and ammonia.

This oxidation is considerably expedited when sewage or water mixed with it percolates through porous strata, and the oxidation is more or less complete as the percolation is more or less thorough. The deeper the well, if surface drainage be excluded, the more complete is the conversion of the dangerous organic matter into the innoxious nitrates; but it can only be said that the danger is lessened by this percolation (which must always be obviously more or less limited in its range) and not done away with, and experience shows that so far as infected water is concerned no amount of possible percolation will remove the poison.

The significance of an excess of nitrates has already been sufficiently dwelt upon, and we have seen that both upon *a priori* grounds and as the result of actual experience, their presence in abnormal quantity is objectionable.

Unpolluted spring water ought to be taken as the standard by which all waters should be judged. The Rivers Pollution Commissioners give* the average composition of unpolluted spring water, calculated from the results obtained from the analysis of 198 samples, as follows :

Parts per 100,000.†

1. Total solid contents, called by the Commissioners, total solid *Impurity* . . 28·2
2. Organic Carbon . . . . . 0·056
   Organic Nitrogen . . . . . 0·013
3. Ammonia . . . . . . 0·001
4. Nitrogen as Nitrates and Nitrites . . 0·383
5. Chlorine . . . . 2·49

Other headings given by the Commissioners, such as " previous sewage or animal contamination," which is calculated from the foregoing figures are not given, as being worse than useless.

The writer's experience confirms that of the Commissioners, and, with reservations to be noticed under the different headings he considers their figures may be conveniently taken as a standard. To take the headings in turn, we come first to "total solid contents." A moderately hard water containing from 20 to 30 parts of total solids in 100,000 parts is, perhaps, the most palatable, though for washing and other

* Sixth Report, p. 425.

† Parts in 100,000 can be converted into grains, per imperial gallon, by multiplying by 7 and then moving the decimal point one place to the left.

domestic purposes no doubt a softer water is desirable. The amount of total solids in different waters is very variable, ranging from as little as less than 3 parts, as in the case of the Loch Katrine water, to as much as 100 and more parts per 100,000.

No. 2.—ORGANIC CARBON AND NITROGEN, or, in other words, organic matter. The quantity given by the Commissioners is a minimum, as measured by Dr. Frankland's process.* Occasionally good water will contain larger quantities of organic matter, but if the proportion of nitrogen as nitrates and chlorine be low, the probability is the organic matter is of vegetable origin and harmless.† It is desirable in such cases to supplement the chemical evidence by examination of the gathering ground of the supply.

3.—AMMONIA.

As with organic matter, so with ammonia : what applies to an excess of the one applies to an excess of the other.

4.—NITROGEN AS NITRATES.

Many waters, such us the surface waters from uncultivated uplands, which supply our large lakes, &c., are sometimes entirely free from nitrates. Analysis shows that in deep unpolluted springs, unpolluted, that is, so far as is possible in an agricultural country where the surface is more or less cultivated, the amount averages from 0·3 to 0·4 parts per 100,000.

---

* For other standards of organic matter see p. 20.

† A few years ago it was found that the water supplied to Bristol was offensive and contained large quantities of ammonia and organic matter, and much alarm was occasioned in consequence. An examination of the water showed that the usual proportion of chlorine and nitrates had not increased, and accordingly it was authoritatively stated that the organic matter was of vegetable origin, and though unpleasant, and to that extent objectionable, it was otherwise harmless. Examination showed that this view was the correct one. The reservoir of the Water Works had become almost choked with confervoid growth, and when this was removed the nuisance ceased.

Springs containing this amount furnish some of our most wholesome waters. When the amount exceeds 0·5 or 0·6 parts, it points significantly to dangerous pollution, and examination of the ground almost invariably shows either that the ground has been heavily manured as in garden ground, or that there is some actual infiltration of sewage.

NITROGEN AS NITRITES.

This should be invariably absent in a good water. It is asserted notwithstanding that in deep wells in the Chalk, nitrites and ammonia are obtained from nitrates by deoxidation, and therefore their presence is not indicative of recent sewage. Even if this reverse action does take place in deep chalk wells as alleged (and there has never been any sufficient proof given of it), it can only take place in the presence of fermenting organic matter, and the significance of the presence of nitrites is therefore as great as if they were formed by oxidation from the organic matter direct. Although our experience of the Chalk is fairly wide, we have only found indications of nitrites in well waters that were certainly polluted, and never in the unpolluted springs of that formation. Nevertheless the opposite view as held by some is here given, and it must be taken for what it is worth.

5.—CHLORINE.

The quantity in good water does not often exceed from 1·7 to 2·3 parts per 100,000, but it must be remembered, as already pointed out, that an excess above this may be entirely derived from the strata through which the water passes.

Bad water has the following characteristics :—When pollution is recent it contains large quantities of organic matter, ammonia, and nitrites; but frequently, especially in shallow wells, the two latter are entirely absent, and the organic matter reduced to a minimum, in which case nitrates will exist in large excess. From 0·9 to 1·1 part per 100,000 nitrogen as nitrates constitutes distinct excess, and no water containing this amount should ever be used for drinking purposes. In the face of the overwhelming evidence that waters containing this amount are dangerous, any exception is so rare that the burden of proof rests entirely with those who assert the contrary. It is not enough to prove that the organic matter is in a minimum quantity, and that ammonia and nitrites are absent ; these characteristics are frequently present in water that has undoubtedly given rise to illness. But it is necessary to prove that the organic matter is harmless, that there are no specific germs or fever poisons present, and that the organic matter will not vary with the rainfall. When these are proved, then, but not till then, can the water be considered safe.

The amount of chlorine in bad water varies from 3 parts, and even less, to several parts per 100,000. Its being present in quantity less than this is not absolute proof of the absence of sewage, and, as has been shown, its presence in excess is not necessarily proof of pollution, but, as a rule, a high figure of nitrogen as nitrates is always accompanied by a high chlorine figure, and *vice versâ*.

The difference between the two standards constitutes the border land in which each case must be decided on its own merits, by the aid of the general considerations already dwelt upon, and where a knowledge of the method of the collection and the surroundings of the source of the supply is invaluable.

The gradations between a good and bad water are infinite, and obviously it is impossible to set up any broad line of demarcation. For example, the quantity of nitrates might be only slightly in excess of the standard, whilst all the other aspects of the water were favourable. Here there would be no justification for positive condemnation, although the experience of the writer convinces him, every day more and more, that even a slight increase of nitrates over the amount given as the standard affords ground for suspicion, and, so far as the public health is concerned, it is a safe axiom to act upon, that a drinking water, like Cæsar's wife, should be above suspicion.

This view of the importance to be attached to an abnormal quantity of nitrates has been formed in spite of a considerable predisposition to a contrary opinion, and has been literally forced upon the writer again and again by the investigation of cases which really leaves no doubt in the matter.

It is highly desirable, however, that those who have had the advantage of being engaged in similar investigations should put their results on record. Probably no men have had a larger experience in inquiring into the conditions, in connection with water supplies, which have given rise to illness than the Medical Inspectors of the Local Government Board, and, in these later days, the Medical Officers of Health to Sanitary Authorities, and it is to their experience that we must look for an authoritative opinion, the digest of accumulated observations, as to the right interpretation of the chemical data supplied by analysts.

It is not pretended that the whole ground has been covered in these pages or the subject exhausted. For instance, the consideration of the examination of water by means of the microscope, and the estimation of phosphates has been purposely avoided, as, in the present state of our knowledge, they afford only additional evidence in cases where the evidence is otherwise already complete, and it has not been thought well to encumber the argument unnecessarily, or distract attention from the main points by the discussion of side issues.

To guide to a correct conclusion has been the object aimed at. The desire has been to state the case fairly and concisely, without sacrificing clearness to brevity, and to give a comprehensive view of general aspects which may enable the careful reader to grasp easily the important and relevant bearings of the question. In this aim the writer hopes he has been successful.

*** For Appendix see next page.

APPENDIX.

Comparative table of cases selected from the Rivers Pollution Commissioners' Sixth Report, in illustration of the foregoing pages, giving the more important features only of the analyses.

Results of analysis expressed in parts per 100,000.*

	Organic Carbon.	Organic Nitrogen.	Ammonia.	Nitrogen as Nitrates and Nitrites.†	Chlorine.
A typically good Spring Water :—					
Eyford Spring, Bath ...	·009	·004	0	·130	1·46
A typically bad Spring Water :—					
Spring in All Saint's Lane, Bristol	·186	·030	·001	4·712	7·10
Waters condemned as polluted by the Rivers Pollution Commissioners, on account of excess of Organic Matter, when in reality they may be good and wholesome.					
Bourne, Lincolnshire ; water supply from deep well	·217	·047	0	0	2·1
Lanark, water supply of	·148	·026	·002	·220	1·8
Eastwood, Notts, from Reservoir supplied by springs	·154	·040	0	·051	1·6

J. & A. CHURCHILL'S

MEDICAL CLASS BOOKS.

ANATOMY.

BRAUNE.—An Atlas of Topographical Ana-
tomy, after Plane Sections of Frozen Bodies. By WILHELM BRAUNE,
Professor of Anatomy in the University of Leipzig. Translated by
EDWARD BELLAMY, F.R.C.S., and Member of the Board of Examiners;
Surgeon to Charing Cross Hospital, and Lecturer on Anatomy in its
School. With 34 Photo-lithographic Plates and 46 Woodcuts. Large
imp. 8vo, 40s.

FLOWER.—Diagrams of the Nerves of the
Human Body, exhibiting their Origin, Divisions, and Connexions, with
their Distribution to the various Regions of the Cutaneous Surface, and
to all the Muscles. By WILLIAM H. FLOWER, F.R.C.S., F.R.S.,
Conservator of the Museum of the Royal College of Surgeons. Second
Edition, containing 6 Plates. Royal 4to, 12s.

GODLEE.—An Atlas of Human Anatomy:
illustrating most of the ordinary Dissections; and many not usually
practised by the Student. By RICKMAN J. GODLEE, M.S., F.R.C.S.,
Assistant-Surgeon to University College Hospital, and Senior
Demonstrator of Anatomy in University College. To be completed in
12 Parts, each containing 4 Coloured Plates, with Explanatory Text.
Parts I. to XI. Imp. 4to, 7s. 6d. each.

HEATH.—Practical Anatomy: a Manual of
Dissections. By CHRISTOPHER HEATH, F.R.C.S., Holme Professor of
Clinical Surgery in University College and Surgeon to the Hospital.
Fourth Edition. With 16 Coloured Plates and 264 Engravings. Crown
8vo, 14s.

NEW BURLINGTON STREET.

ANATOMY—*continued.*

HOLDEN.—Human Osteology : comprising a
Description of the Bones, with Delineations of the Attachments of the
Muscles, the General and Microscopical Structure of Bone and its
Development. By LUTHER HOLDEN, F.R.C.S., Senior Surgeon to St.
Bartholomew's and the Foundling Hospitals, and ALBAN DORAN,
F.R.C.S., late Anatomical, now Pathological, Assistant to the Museum
of the Royal College of Surgeons. Fifth Edition. With 61 Lithographic
Plates and 89 Engravings. Royal 8vo, 16s.

By the same Author.

A Manual of the Dissection of the
Human Body. Fourth Edition. Revised by the Author and
JOHN LANGTON, F.R.C.S., Assistant Surgeon and Lecturer on
Anatomy at St. Bartholomew's Hospital. With Engravings.
8vo, 16s.

ALSO,

Landmarks, Medical and Surgical. Second
Edition. 8vo, 3s. 6d.

MORRIS.—The Anatomy of the Joints of Man.
By HENRY MORRIS, M.A., F.R.C.S., Surgeon to, and Lecturer on Ana-
tomy and Practical Surgery at, the Middlesex Hospital. With 44
Plates (19 Coloured) and Engravings. 8vo, 16s.

WAGSTAFFE.—The Student's Guide to Human
Osteology. By WM. WARWICK WAGSTAFFE, F.R.C.S., Assistant-
Surgeon to, and Lecturer on Anatomy at, St. Thomas's Hospital.
With 23 Plates and 66 Engravings. Fcap. 8vo, 10s. 6d.

WILSON — BUCHANAN — CLARK.— Wilson's
Anatomist's Vade-Mecum: a System of Human Anatomy. Ninth
Edition, by GEORGE BUCHANAN, Professor of Clinical Surgery in the
University of Glasgow, and HENRY E. CLARK, M.R.C.S , Lecturer on
Anatomy in the Glasgow Royal Infirmary School of Medicine. With
371 Engravings. Crown 8vo, 14s.

Anatomical Remembrancer (the); or, Complete Pocket Anatomist. Eighth Edition. 32mo, 3s. 6d.

NEW BURLINGTON STREET.

BOTANY.

BENTLEY.—A Manual of Botany. By Robert
BENTLEY, F.L.S., Professor of Botany in King's College and to the
Pharmaceutical Society. With 1138 Engravings. Fourth Edition.
Crown 8vo. [*In preparation.*

BENTLEY AND TRIMEN.—Medicinal Plants:
being descriptions, with original Figures, of the Principal Plants
employed in Medicine, and an account of their Properties and Uses.
By ROBERT BENTLEY, F.L.S., and HENRY TRIMEN, M.B., F.L.S., British
Museum, and Lecturer on Botany at St. Mary's Hospital Medical
School. In 4 Vols., large 8vo, with 306 Coloured Plates, bound in
half morocco, gilt edges, £11 11s.

CHEMISTRY.

BERNAYS.—Notes for Students in Chemistry;
being a Syllabus of Chemistry compiled mainly from the Manuals of
Fownes-Watts, Miller, Wurz, and Schorlemmer. By ALBERT J. BERNAYS,
Ph.D., Professor of Chemistry at St. Thomas's Hospital, Examiner
in Chemistry at the Royal College of Physicians of London. Sixth
Edition. Fcap. 8vo, 3s. 6d.

By the same Author.

Skeleton Notes on Analytical Chemistry,
for Students in Medicine. Fcap. 8vo, 2s. 6d.

BLOXAM.—Chemistry, Inorganic and Organic;
with Experiments. By CHARLES L. BLOXAM, Professor of Chemistry in
King's College. Fourth Edition. With nearly 300 Engravings. 8vo, 16s.

By the same Author.

Laboratory Teaching; or, Progressive
Exercises in Practical Chemistry. Fourth Edition. With 83
Engravings. Crown 8vo, 5s. 6d.

BOWMAN AND BLOXAM.—Practical Chemistry,
including Analysis. By JOHN E. BOWMAN, formerly Professor of
Practical Chemistry in King's College, and CHARLES L. BLOXAM,
Professor of Chemistry in King's College. With 98 Engravings.
Seventh Edition. Fcap. 8vo, 6s. 6d.

CHEMISTRY—*continued.*

CLOWES.—Practical Chemistry and Qualitative Inorganic Analysis. An Elementary Treatise specially adapted for use in the Laboratories of Schools and Colleges, and by Beginners. By FRANK CLOWES, D.Sc., Senior Science Master at the High School, Newcastle-under-Lyme. Third Edition. With 47 Engravings. Post 8vo, 7s. 6d.

FOWNES AND WATTS.—Physical and Inorganic Chemistry. Twelfth Edition. By GEORGE FOWNES, F.R.S., and HENRY WATTS, B.A., F.R.S. With 154 Engravings, and Coloured Plate of Spectra. Crown 8vo, 8s. 6d.

By the same Authors.

Chemistry of Carbon - Compounds, or
Organic Chemistry. Twelfth Edition. With Engravings. Crown 8vo, 10s.

GALLOWAY.—A Manual of Qualitative Analysis. By ROBERT GALLOWAY, late Professor of Applied Chemistry in the Royal College of Science for Ireland. Fifth Edition. With Engravings. Post 8vo, 8s. 6d.

LUFF.—An Introduction to the Study of Chemistry. Specially designed for Medical and Pharmaceutical Students. By A. P. LUFF, F.I.C., F.C.S., Lecturer on Chemistry in the Central School of Chemistry and Pharmacy. Crown 8vo, 2s. 6d.

VACHER.—A Primer of Chemistry, including Analysis. By ARTHUR VACHER. 18mo, 1s.

VALENTIN.—Introduction to Inorganic Chemistry. By WILLIAM G. VALENTIN, F.C.S. Third Edition. With 82 Engravings. 8vo, 6s. 6d.

By the same Author.

A Course of Qualitative Chemical Analysis.
Fifth Edition by W. R. HODGKINSON, Ph.D. (Würzburg), Demonstrator of Practical Chemistry in the Science Training Schools. With Engravings. 8vo, 7s. 6d.

ALSO,

Chemical Tables for the Lecture-room and
Laboratory. In Five large Sheets, 5s. 6d.

CHILDREN, DISEASES OF.

ELLIS.—A Practical Manual of the Diseases of Children. By EDWARD ELLIS, M.D., late Senior Physician to the Victoria Hospital for Sick Children. With a Formulary. Fourth Edition. Crown 8vo. [*In preparation.*]

SMITH. — Clinical Studies of Disease in Children. By EUSTACE SMITH, M.D., F.R.C.P., Physician to H.M. the King of the Belgians, and to the East London Hospital for Children. Post 8vo, 7s. 6d.

By the same Author.

On the Wasting Diseases of Infants and Children. Third Edition. Post 8vo, 8s. 6d.

STEINER.—Compendium of Children's Diseases; a Handbook for Practitioners and Students. By JOHANN STEINER, M.D. Translated from the Second German Edition, by LAWSON TAIT, F.R.C.S., Surgeon to the Birmingham Hospital for Women, &c. 8vo, 12s. 6d.

DENTISTRY.

SEWILL.—The Student's Guide to Dental Anatomy and Surgery. By HENRY E. SEWILL, M.R.C.S., L.D.S., late Dental Surgeon to the West London Hospital. With 77 Engravings. Fcap. 8vo, 5s. 6d.

SMITH.—Handbook of Dental Anatomy and Surgery. For the Use of Students and Practitioners. By JOHN SMITH, M.D., F.R.S.E., Dental Surgeon to the Royal Infirmary, Edinburgh. Second Edition. Fcap. 8vo, 4s. 6d.

STOCKEN.—Elements of Dental Materia Medica and Therapeutics, with Pharmacopœia. By JAMES STOCKEN, L.D.S.R.C.S., late Lecturer on Dental Materia Medica and Therapeutics and Dental Surgeon to the National Dental Hospital. Second Edition. Fcap. 8vo, 6s. 6d.

DENTISTRY—*continued.*

TAFT.—A Practical Treatise on Operative
Dentistry. By JONATHAN TAFT, D.D.S., Professor of Operative Surgery
in the Ohio College of Dental Surgery. Third Edition. With 134
Engravings. 8vo, 18s.

TOMES (C. S.).—Manual of Dental Anatomy,
Human and Comparative. By CHARLES S. TOMES, M.A., M.R.C.S.,
Lecturer on Anatomy and Physiology at the Dental Hospital of London.
With 179 Engravings. Crown 8vo, 10s. 6d.

TOMES (J. and C. S.).—A Manual of Dental
Surgery. By JOHN TOMES, M.R.C.S., F.R.S., Consulting Surgeon-Dentist
to Middlesex Hospital; and CHARLES S. TOMES, M.A., M.R.C.S.,
Lecturer on Anatomy and Physiology at the Dental Hospital of London. Second Edition. With 262 Engravings. Fcap. 8vo, 14s.

EAR, DISEASES OF.

BURNETT.—The Ear: its Anatomy, Physio-
logy, and Diseases. A Practical Treatise for the Use of Medical
Students and Practitioners. By CHARLES H. BURNETT, M.D., Aural
Surgeon to the Presbyterian Hospital, Philadelphia. With 87 Engravings. 8vo, 18s.

DALBY.—On Diseases and Injuries of the Ear.
By WILLIAM B. DALBY, F.R.C.S., Aural Surgeon to, and Lecturer on
Aural Surgery at, St. George's Hospital. With Engravings. Fcap. 8vo,
6s. 6d.

JONES.—A Practical Treatise on Aural Sur-
gery. By H. MACNAUGHTON JONES, M.D., Professor of the Queen's
University in Ireland, Surgeon to the Cork Ophthalmic and Aural Hospital. With 46 Engravings. Crown 8vo, 5s.

By the same Author.

Atlas of the Diseases of the Membrana
Tympani. In Coloured Plates, containing 59 Figures. With Explanatory Text. Crown 4to, 21s.

FORENSIC MEDICINE.

OGSTON.—Lectures on Medical Jurisprudence.
By FRANCIS OGSTON, M.D., Professor of Medical Jurisprudence and Medical Logic in the University of Aberdeen. Edited by FRANCIS OGSTON, Jun., M.D., Assistant to the Professor of Medical Jurisprudence and Lecturer on Practical Toxicology in the University of Aberdeen. With 12 Plates. 8vo, 18s.

TAYLOR.—The Principles and Practice of
Medical Jurisprudence. By ALFRED S. TAYLOR, M.D., F.R.S., late Professor of Medical Jurisprudence to Guy's Hospital. Second Edition. With 189 Engravings. 2 Vols. 8vo, 31s. 6d.

By the same Author.

A Manual of Medical Jurisprudence.
Tenth Edition. With 55 Engravings. Crown 8vo, 14s.

ALSO,

On Poisons, in relation to Medical Jurisprudence and Medicine. Third Edition. With 104 Engravings. Crown 8vo, 16s.

WOODMAN AND TIDY.—A Handy-Book of
Forensic Medicine and Toxicology. By W. BATHURST WOODMAN, M.D., F.R.C.P.; and C. MEYMOTT TIDY, M.B., Professor of Chemistry and of Medical Jurisprudence, &c., at the London Hospital. With 8 Lithographic Plates and 116 Wood Engravings. 8vo, 31s. 6d.

HYGIENE.

WILSON.—A Handbook of Hygiene and Sanitary Science. By GEORGE WILSON, M.A., M.D., Medical Officer of Health for Mid Warwickshire. Fourth Edition. With Engravings. Crown 8vo, 10s. 6d.

HYGIENE—*continued.*

PARKES.—A Manual of Practical Hygiene.
By EDMUND A. PARKES, M.D., F.R.S. Fifth Edition by F. DE CHAUMONT, M.D., F.R.S., Professor of Military Hygiene in the Army Medical School. With 9 Plates and 112 Engravings. 8vo, 18s.

By the same Author.

Public Health: being a Concise Sketch of
the Sanitary Considerations connected with the Land, with Cities, Villages, Houses, and Individuals. Revised by WILLIAM AITKEN, M.D., F.R.S., Professor of Pathology in the Army Medical School. Crown 8vo, 2s. 6d.

MATERIA MEDICA AND THERAPEUTICS.

BINZ AND SPARKS.—The Elements of Thera-
peutics: a Clinical Guide to the Action of Medicines. By C. BINZ, M.D., Professor of Pharmacology in the University of Bonn. Translated from the Fifth German Edition, and Edited with Additions, in conformity with the British and American Pharmacopœias, by EDWARD I. SPARKS, M.A., M.B. Oxon., F.R.C.P. Lond. Crown 8vo, 8s. 6d.

ROYLE AND HARLEY.—A Manual of Materia
Medica and Therapeutics. By J. FORBES ROYLE, M.D., F.R.S., formerly Professor of Materia Medica in King's College; and JOHN HARLEY, M.D., F.R.C.P., Physician to, and Joint Lecturer on Clinical Medicine at, St. Thomas's Hospital. Sixth Edition. With 139 Engravings. Crown 8vo, 15s.

THOROWGOOD.—The Student's Guide to
Materia Medica. By JOHN C. THOROWGOOD, M.D., F.R.C.P., Lecturer on Materia Medica at the Middlesex Hospital. With Engravings. Fcap. 8vo, 6s. 6d.

WARING.—A Manual of Practical Therapeu-
tics. By EDWARD J. WARING, M.D., F.R.C.P., Retired Surgeon H.M. Indian Army. Third Edition. Fcap. 8vo, 12s. 6d.

MEDICINE.

BARCLAY.—A Manual of Medical Diagnosis.
By A. WHYTE BARCLAY, M.D., F.R.C.P., Physician to, and Lecturer on Medicine at, St. George's Hospital. Third Edition. Fcap. 8vo, 10s. 6d.

BARLOW.—A Manual of the Practice of
Medicine. By HILARO BARLOW, M.D., formerly Senior Physician to Guy's Hospital. Second Edition. Fcap. 8vo, 7s. 6d.

CHARTERIS.—The Student's Guide to the
Practice of Medicine. By MATTHEW CHARTERIS, M.D., Professor of Practice of Medicine, Anderson's College ; Physician and Lecturer on Clinical Medicine, Royal Infirmary, Glasgow. With Engravings on Copper and Wood. Second Edition. Fcap. 8vo, 6s. 6d.

FENWICK.—The Student's Guide to Medical
Diagnosis. By SAMUEL FENWICK, M.D., F.R.C.P., Physician to the London Hospital. Fourth Edition. With 106 Engravings. Fcap. 8vo, 6s. 6d.

By the same Author.
The Student's Outlines of Medical Treat-
· ment. Fcap. 8vo, 7s.

FLINT.—Clinical Medicine : a Systematic Trea-
tise on the Diagnosis and Treatment of Disease. By AUSTIN FLINT, M.D., Professor of the Principles and Practice of Medicine, &c., in Bellevue Hospital Medical College. 8vo, 20s.

By the same Author.
A Manual of Percussion and Auscultation ;
of the Physical Diagnosis of Diseases of the Lungs and Heart, and of Thoracic Aneurism. Post 8vo, 6s. 6d.

HALL.—Synopsis of the Diseases of the Larynx,
Lungs, and Heart : comprising Dr. Edwards' Tables on the Examination of the Chest. With Alterations and Additions. By F. DE HAVILLAND HALL, M.D., Assistant-Physician to the Westminster Hospital. Royal 8vo, 2s. 6d.

MIDWIFERY.

BARNES.—Lectures on Obstetric Operations,
including the Treatment of Hæmorrhage, and forming a Guide to the
Management of Difficult Labour. By ROBERT BARNES, M.D., F.R.C.P.,
Obstetric Physician to, and Lecturer on Diseases of Women, &c., at St.
George's Hospital. Third Edition. With 124 Engravings. 8vo, 18s.

CLAY.—The Complete Handbook of Obstetric
Surgery; or, Short Rules of Practice in every Emergency, from the
Simplest to the most formidable Operations connected with the Science
of Obstetricy. By CHARLES CLAY, M.D., late Senior Surgeon to, and
Lecturer on Midwifery at, St. Mary's Hospital, Manchester. Third
Edition. With 91 Engravings. Fcap. 8vo, 6s. 6d.

RAMSBOTHAM.—The Principles and Practice
of Obstetric Medicine and Surgery. By FRANCIS H. RAMSBOTHAM, M.D.,
formerly Obstetric Physician to the London Hospital. Fifth Edition.
Illustrated with 120 Plates, forming one thick handsome volume. 8vo,
22s.

ROBERTS.—The Student's Guide to the Practice
of Midwifery. By D. LLOYD ROBERTS, M.D., F.R.C.P., Physician to
St. Mary's Hospital, Manchester. Second Edition. With 96 Engravings. Fcap. 8vo, 7s.

SCHROEDER.—A Manual of Midwifery; includ-
ing the Pathology of Pregnancy and the Puerperal State. By KARL
SCHROEDER, M.D., Professor of Midwifery in the University of Erlangen.
Translated by CHARLES H. CARTER, M.D. With Engravings. 8vo,
12s. 6d.

SWAYNE.—Obstetric Aphorisms for the Use of
Students commencing Midwifery Practice. By JOSEPH G. SWAYNE,
M.D., Lecturer on Midwifery at the Bristol School of Medicine. Seventh
Edition. With Engravings. Fcap. 8vo, 3s. 6d.

NEW BURLINGTON STREET.

MICROSCOPY.

CARPENTER.—The Microscope and its Revelations. By WILLIAM B. CARPENTER, C.B., M.D., F.R.S., late Registrar to the University of London. Sixth Edition. With more than 500 Engravings. Crown 8vo. : `[In preparation.`

MARSH.—Section-Cutting : a Practical Guide to the Preparation and Mounting of Sections for the Microscope, special prominence being given to the subject of Animal Sections. By Dr. SYLVESTER MARSH. With Engravings. Fcap. 8vo, 2s. 6d.

MARTIN.—A Manual of Microscopic Mounting. By JOHN H. MARTIN, Member of the Society of Public Analysts, &c. Second Edition. With several Plates and 144 Engravings. 8vo, 7s. 6d.

WYTHE.—The Microscopist : a Manual of Microscopy and Compendium of the Microscopic Sciences, Micro-Mineralogy, Micro-Chemistry, Biology, Histology, and Pathological Histology. By J. H. WYTHE, A.M., M.D., Professor of Microscopy and Biology in the San Francisco Medical College. Third Edition. With 205 Illustrations. Royal 8vo, 18s.

OPHTHALMOLOGY.

HIGGENS.—Hints on Ophthalmic Out-Patient Practice. By CHARLES HIGGENS, F.R.C.S., Ophthalmic Assistant-Surgeon to, and Lecturer on Ophthalmology at, Guy's Hospital. Second Edition. Fcap. 8vo, 3s.

JONES.—A Manual of the Principles and Practice of Ophthalmic Medicine and Surgery. By T. WHARTON JONES, F.R.C.S., F.R.S., Ophthalmic Surgeon and Professor of Ophthalmology to University College Hospital. Third Edition. With 9 Coloured Plates and 173 Engravings. Fcap. 8vo, 12s. 6d.

MACNAMARA.—A Manual of the Diseases of the Eye. By CHARLES MACNAMARA, F.R.C.S., Surgeon to Westminster Hospital. Third Edition. With 7 Coloured Plates and 52 Engravings. Fcap. 8vo, 12s. 6d.

OPHTHALMOLOGY—*continued.*

NETTLESHIP.—The Student's Guide to Diseases
of the Eye. By EDWARD NETTLESHIP, F.R.C.S., Ophthalmic Surgeon
to, and Lecturer on Ophthalmic Surgery at, St. Thomas's Hospital.
With 48 Engravings. Fcap. 8vo, 7s. 6d.

WELLS.—A Treatise on the Diseases of the
Eye. By J. SOELBERG WELLS, F.R.C.S., late Ophthalmic Surgeon to
King's College Hospital, and Professor of Ophthalmology at King's Col-
lege. With Coloured Plates and Engravings. Third Edition. 8vo, 25s.

PATHOLOGY.

JONES AND SIEVEKING.—A Manual of Patho-
logical Anatomy. By C. HANDFIELD JONES, M.B., F.R.S., Physician to
St. Mary's Hospital, and EDWARD H. SIEVEKING, M.D., F.R.C.P., Physi-
cian to St. Mary's Hospital. Second Edition. Edited by J. F. PAYNE,
M.B., Assistant-Physician and Lecturer on General Pathology at St.
Thomas's Hospital. With 195 Engravings. Crown 8vo, 16s.

VIRCHOW. — Post-Mortem Examinations: a
Description and Explanation of the Method of Performing them,
with especial reference to Medico-Legal Practice. By Professor
RUDOLPH VIRCHOW, Berlin Charité Hospital. Translated by Dr. T. B.
SMITH. Second Edition, with 4 Plates. Fcap. 8vo, 3s. 6d.

WILKS AND MOXON.—Lectures on Pathologi-
cal Anatomy. By SAMUEL WILKS, M.D., F.R.S., Physician to, and
Lecturer on Medicine at, Guy's Hospital; and WALTER MOXON, M.D.,
F.R.C.P., Physician to, and Lecturer on Clinical Medicine at, Guy's
Hospital. Second Edition. With 5 Steel Plates. 8vo, 18s.

PSYCHOLOGY.

BUCKNILL AND TUKE.—A Manual of Psycho-
logical Medicine: containing the Lunacy Laws, Nosology, Ætiology,
Statistics, Description, Diagnosis, Pathology, and Treatment of Insanity,
with an Appendix of Cases. By JOHN C. BUCKNILL, M.D., F.R.S.,
and D. HACK TUKE, M.D., F.R.C.P. Fourth Edition, with 12 Plates
(30 Figures). 8vo, 25s.

PHYSIOLOGY.

CARPENTER.—Principles of Human Physio-
logy. With 3 Steel Plates and 371 Engravings. By WILLIAM B.
CARPENTER, C.B., M.D., F.R.S., late Registrar to the University of
London. Eighth Edition. Edited by Mr. Henry Power. 8vo, 31s. 6d.

By the same Author.

A Manual of Physiology. With upwards
of 250 Illustrations. Fifth Edition. Edited by P. H. PYE-SMITH,
M.D., F.R.C.P. Crown 8vo. [*In preparation.*

DALTON.—A Treatise on Human Physiology :
designed for the use of Students and Practitioners of Medicine. By
JOHN C. DALTON, M.D., Professor of Physiology and Hygiene in the
College of Physicians and Surgeons, New York. Sixth Edition. With
316 Engravings. Royal 8vo, 20s.

FREY.—The Histology and Histo-Chemistry of
Man. A Treatise on the Elements of Composition and Structure of the
Human Body. By HEINRICH FREY, Professor of Medicine in Zurich.
Translated from the Fourth German Edition, by ARTHUR E. BARKER,
Assistant-Surgeon to the University College Hospital. With 608
Engravings. 8vo, 21s.

FULTON.—A Text-Book of Physiology, includ-
ing Histology. By J. FULTON, M.D., Professor of Physiology and
Sanitary Science in Trinity Medical College, Toronto ; Surgeon to the
Toronto General Hospital. Second Edition, with 151 Engravings.
8vo, 15s.

RUTHERFORD.—Outlines of Practical Histo-
logy. By WILLIAM RUTHERFORD, M.D., F.R.S., Professor of the Insti-
tutes of Medicine in the University of Edinburgh ; Examiner in
Physiology in the University of London. Second Edition. With 63
Engravings. Crown 8vo (with additional leaves for Notes), 6s.

SANDERSON.—Handbook for the Physiological
Laboratory : containing an Exposition of the fundamental facts of the
Science, with explicit Directions for their demonstration. By J. BURDON
SANDERSON, M.D., F.R.S., Professor and Superintendent of the Brown
Institution ; E. KLEIN, M.D., F.R.S., Assistant-Professor in the Brown
Institution ; MICHAEL FOSTER, M.D., F.R.S., Prælector of Physiology
at Trinity College, Cambridge ; and T. LAUDER BRUNTON, M.D., F.R.S.,
Lecturer on Materia Medica at St. Bartholomew's Hospital Medical
College. 2 Vols., with 123 Plates. 8vo, 24s.

SURGERY.

BRYANT. — A Manual for the Practice of Surgery. By THOMAS BRYANT, F.R.C.S., Surgeon to, and Lecturer on Surgery at, Guy's Hospital. Third Edition. With 672 Engravings (nearly all original, many being coloured). 2 vols. Crown 8vo, 28s.

BELLAMY.—The Student's Guide to Surgical Anatomy; a Description of the more important Surgical Regions of the Human Body, and an Introduction to Operative Surgery. By EDWARD BELLAMY, F.R.C.S., and Member of the Board of Examiners; Surgeon to, and Lecturer on Anatomy at, Charing Cross Hospital. Second Edition. With 76 Engravings. Fcap. 8vo, 7s.

CLARK AND WAGSTAFFE. — Outlines of Surgery and Surgical Pathology. By F. LE GROS CLARK, F.R.C.S., F.R.S., Consulting Surgeon to St. Thomas's and the Great Northern Hospitals. Second Edition. Revised and expanded by the Author, assisted by W. W. WAGSTAFFE, F.R.C.S., Assistant-Surgeon to St. Thomas's Hospital. 8vo, 10s. 6d.

DRUITT. — The Surgeon's Vade-Mecum; a Manual of Modern Surgery. By ROBERT DRUITT, F.R.C.S. Eleventh Edition. With 369 Engravings. Fcap. 8vo, 14s.

FERGUSSON.—A System of Practical Surgery. By Sir WILLIAM FERGUSSON, Bart., F.R.C.S., F.R.S., late Surgeon and Professor of Clinical Surgery to King's College Hospital. With 463 Engravings. Fifth Edition. 8vo, 21s.

HEATH.—A Manual of Minor Surgery and Bandaging, for the use of House-Surgeons, Dressers, and Junior Practitioners. By CHRISTOPHER HEATH, F.R.C.S., Holme Professor of Clinical Surgery in University College and Surgeon to the Hospital. Sixth Edition. With 115 Engravings. Fcap. 8vo. 5s. 6d.

By the same Author.

A Course of Operative Surgery: with Twenty Plates drawn from Nature by M. LÉVEILLÉ, and Coloured by hand under his direction. Large 8vo, 40s.

ALSO,

The Student's Guide to Surgical Diagnosis. Fcap. 8vo, 6s. 6d.

SURGERY—*continued.*

MAUNDER.—Operative Surgery. By Charles
F. MAUNDER, F.R.C.S., late Surgeon to, and Lecturer on Surgery at,
the London Hospital. Second Edition. With 164 Engravings. Post
8vo, 6s.

PIRRIE.—The Principles and Practice of
Surgery. By WILLIAM PIRRIE, F.R.S.E., Professor of Surgery in the
University of Aberdeen. Third Edition. With 490 Engravings. 8vo, 28s.

TERMINOLOGY.

DUNGLISON.—Medical Lexicon : a Dictionary
of Medical Science, containing a concise Explanation of its various
Subjects and Terms, with Accentuation, Etymology, Synonymes, &c.
By ROBLEY DUNGLISON, M.D. New Edition, thoroughly revised by
RICHARD J. DUNGLISON, M.D. Royal 8vo, 28s.

MAYNE.—A Medical Vocabulary : being an
Explanation of all Terms and Phrases used in the various Depart-
ments of Medical Science and Practice, giving their Derivation, Meaning,
Application, and Pronunciation. By ROBERT G. MAYNE, M.D., LL.D.,
and JOHN MAYNE, M.D., L.R.C.S.E. Fourth Edition. Fcap. 8vo, 10s.

WOMEN, DISEASES OF.

BARNES.—A Clinical History of the Medical
and Surgical Diseases of Women. By ROBERT BARNES, M.D., F.R.C.P.,
Obstetric Physician to, and Lecturer on Diseases of Women, &c., at, St.
George's Hospital. Second Edition. With 181 Engravings. 8vo, 28s.

DUNCAN.—Clinical Lectures on the Diseases
of Women. By J. MATTHEWS DUNCAN, M.D., Obstetric Physician to
St. Bartholomew's Hospital. 8vo, 8s.

EMMET. — The Principles and Practice of
Gynæcology. By THOMAS ADDIS EMMET, M.D., Surgeon to the
Woman's Hospital of the State of New York. With 130 Engravings.
Royal 8vo, 24s.

WOMEN, DISEASES OF—*continued*.

GALABIN.—The Student's Guide to the Diseases of Women. By ALFRED L. GALABIN, M.D., F.R.C.P., Assistant Obstetric Physician and Joint Lecturer on Obstetric Medicine to Guy's Hospital. With 63 Engravings. Fcap. 8vo, 7s. 6d.

SMITH.—Practical Gynæcology: a Handbook of the Diseases of Women. By HEYWOOD SMITH, M.D., Physician to the Hospital for Women, and to the British Lying-in Hospital. With Engravings. Crown 8vo, 5s. 6d.

WEST AND DUNCAN.—Lectures on the Diseases of Women. By CHARLES WEST, M.D., F.R.C.P. Fourth Edition. Revised and in part re-written by the Author, with numerous additions, by J. MATTHEWS DUNCAN, M.D., Obstetric Physician to St. Bartholomew's Hospital. 8vo, 16s.

ZOOLOGY.

BRADLEY.—Manual of Comparative Anatomy and Physiology. By S. MESSENGER BRADLEY, F.R.C.S., Lecturer on Practical Surgery in Owen's College, Manchester. Third Edition. With 61 Engravings. Post 8vo, 6s. 6d.

CHAUVEAU AND FLEMING.—The Comparative Anatomy of the Domesticated Animals. By A. CHAUVEAU, Professor at the Lyons Veterinary School; and GEORGE FLEMING, Veterinary Surgeon, Royal Engineers. With 450 Engravings. 8vo, 31s. 6d.

HUXLEY.—Manual of the Anatomy of Invertebrated Animals. By THOMAS H. HUXLEY, LL.D., F.R.S. With 156 Engravings. Fcap. 8vo, 16s.

By the same Author.

Manual of the Anatomy of Vertebrated Animals. With 110 Engravings. Post 8vo, 12s.

WILSON.—The Student's Guide to Zoology: a Manual of the Principles of Zoological Science. By ANDREW WILSON, Lecturer on Natural History, Edinburgh. With Engravings. Fcap. 8vo, 6s. 6d.

www.ingramcontent.com/pod-product-compliance
Lightning Source LLC
Chambersburg PA
CBHW032134080426
42733CB00008B/1062